"Try CoQ10 . . . you'll all feel better!"

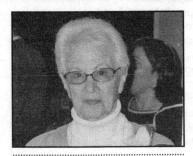

Lucy O.
Eugene, Oregon

"I started using CoQ10 five years ago. After reading about how it might help support heart health, I decided to give it a try. It helped me in lots of ways. I found I was working almost as good as when I was much younger. You see, I am approaching 90. I felt like dancing around the house and swinging it. My outlook on life seemed better.

Before taking CoQ10 I felt tired and sluggish. Now I can once again look at life with calmness and even flirt a little. More pep, more energy, more eager to try new things and make my dreams come true.

I have recommended CoQ10 to all my friends when they asked me why I was so energized. A man recently shook my hand and said to everyone at the party, 'What a grip for a woman who's going to be 90.' I replied, 'Try CoQ10… you'll all feel better!'"

"[CoQ10] has changed my life!"

"'Where should we hike this weekend? Do you want to take a bike ride with me? Who wants to come with me to walk the dogs?' These are a few of the questions I ask my family since I've been taking CoQ10. It has changed my life!

Before taking CoQ10 I could function, but had to content myself with just getting through the day. That is no way to live.

I consulted an herbalist/registered nurse and she suggested I take CoQ10. What a difference it made – and continues to make. I recommend it to friends who

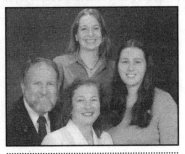

Denise P.
Laurel, Maryland

complain about losing their zest for living. For myself, I now look forward to each day. I may not bound out of bed each morning, but I greet each day with a big smile wondering what adventures I'll share with my family and friends. Can I engage in walking, hiking and biking? Yes I can – with CoQ10!"

1

Vibrant Life Publishing, Inc.
1427 East Hillsboro Blvd.
Suite 425
Deerfield Beach, Florida 33441
1-877-778-5178
www.vibrantlifepublishing.com

Copyright© 2009 by Vibrant Life Publishing, Inc.

ISBN: 978-0-9815547-2-3

Printed in the USA

TABLE OF CONTENTS

By Gian Paolo Littarru, MD

This book represents an admirable approach in explaining to the person on the street how Coenzyme Q10 works and how one feels when taking CoQ10. The simple, yet incisive language which the author uses is not, of course, a rigorous scientific one, but always tries to be supported by the scientific evidence which lies behind the mechanisms of CoQ10 activity.

A remarkable aspect of this book is constituted by the testimonials of people who have experienced the benefits of CoQ10. Even though anecdotal observations cannot be cited in a scientific work, they may reveal real effects which should not be ignored. Sometimes feeling better can be one of the signs of improved biochemical activity, which we usually measure by monitoring molecular and physiological mechanisms.

People might wonder how CoQ10 can work in so many different fields: its deep involvement in providing energy to all the cells and its antioxidant protection make it an essential molecule for the many tasks of the different tissues and organs of our body and this book gives a good idea of how all this occurs.

Dr. Gian Paolo Littarru is one of the world's foremost experts on Coenzyme Q10. He is the author of numerous papers on basic and applied aspects of Coenzyme Q10 and of some books, including "Energy and Defense: Facts and Perspectives on Coenzyme Q10 in Biology and Medicine" (Casa Editrice Scientifica Internazionale). Early in his career, Dr. Littarru studied under Dr. Karl Folkers, the pioneer in the clinical use of CoQ10. Dr. Littarru is a past research associate of Cellular Biochemistry at the University of Texas and is presently a Professor of Biochemistry at the University of Ancona, Italy. Dr. Littarru's expertise in the CoQ10 field is exemplified by his position as Chairman of the International Coenzyme Q10 Association (ICQA), a non-profit organization dedicated to promoting research and educational activities related to CoQ10. To learn more about the ICQA, please visit www.icqa.org.

The Omnipresent Supernutrient

"Five years ago, at age 69, while teaching music in northern California public schools, I was faced with one of life's little surprises: I had to undergo heart surgery. After surgery I felt like a zombie. Enter CoQ10: within two weeks, I noticed an increase in my energy and well-being. By the fall I was back in the teaching saddle again, resuming my full-time position. Although I was assigned a challenging schedule traveling between three middle schools with no break, I did not miss one day of school all year long!

Now, at almost age 74, I continue to teach nearly 200 students and maintain a full-time teaching position while traveling to 12 elementary schools each

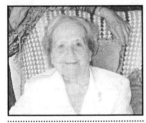

Mary S.
San Francisco, CA

week. My colleagues joke about how I have more energy than they do even though they are 16 to 20 years younger! Now I share my CoQ10 secret with them and my family. Even my husband has become a believer since taking CoQ10, and claims that he requires fewer hours of sleep, yet awakes more refreshed.

I regard CoQ10 as a 'miracle substance' and consider it my most valuable supplement because of the incredible strength and energy it gives me."

NATURE'S SUBLIME DESIGN

What does it mean when Nature places a substance in practically every single cell in the human body? Perhaps more importantly, what happens when this substance starts to disappear from our cells? In Nature's sublime design, anything that is present in nearly every single cell in the human body must possess remarkable significance – or else it would not be there.

Coenzyme Q10 – also known as CoQ10 or ubiquinone – is *the* ubiquitous supernutrient. The word "ubiquinone" is derived from the word "ubiquitous" – and true to its name, CoQ10 is present in practically every cell in the human body. Here, CoQ10 performs two vital functions:

- CoQ10 is vital for energy production throughout the body[1]
- CoQ10 as **Ubiquinol** provides powerful antioxidant protection[2]

From these two actions, CoQ10 delivers nutritional support that expands to encompass whole-body health. The energy and protection that CoQ10 promotes on a cellular level are mirrored in overall vitality – the end result is seen in a diversity of health-boosting, life-sustaining benefits.

Since CoQ10 is necessary for cellular energy, it's no surprise that it is highly regarded for promoting peak vitality. Many who struggle with fatigue report that CoQ10 is an amazing recharger. CoQ10 is also famous for supporting cardiovascular health. Numerous studies have investigated CoQ10's impact on the heart, amassing promising evidence for benefits to blood pressure, heart health and more.

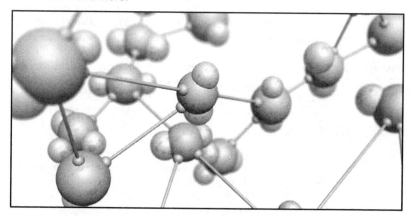

Further, CoQ10's close relationship with cellular health may promote many more health benefits. CoQ10 has been clinically tested for its impact on:

- Tinnitus (ringing ears)
- Diabetes
- Migraine Headaches
- Gum Disease
- Exercise Performance
- Immune Disorders
- Asthma
- Neurodegenerative Problems

Anecdotal evidence, such as the stories appearing throughout this book, reveal even more exciting potential CoQ10 benefits – many who take supplemental CoQ10 find themselves enjoying improved overall quality of life that is often described as a "miraculous" change.

The bad news: Many Americans face declining CoQ10 levels. The statin drugs that over 20 million Americans take for heart problems and high cholesterol are known to deplete CoQ10 in the body. Aging, unhealthy diets, toxins and stress can also diminish CoQ10 levels. **Some experts believe that this CoQ10 decline is partly responsible for age-related health problems.**[3]

CoQ10 supplementation presents a potential solution to diminished CoQ10 levels. But to best achieve CoQ10's support for peak well-being, it is helpful to have a better understanding of the story behind the supernutrient. Read on to learn about CoQ10 and its active form, Ubiquinol.

The Ubiquinol Advantage

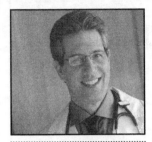

Dennis Goodman, MD, FACP
New York, NY
Integrative Cardiologist

"I recommend Ubiquinol in my practice because it provides the optimal benefits of CoQ10 in a form more easily assimilated in the body. Many of the medications prescribed by cardiologists, like statins and other cholesterol-lowering drugs, reduce CoQ10 levels in the body – which actually puts patients at higher risk! New research shows that Ubiquinol supplementation can yield up to a 3-fold increase in Ubiquinol levels in cardiovascular patients. In addition, it dramatically improves the heart's pumping ability! I believe we've just touched the surface in terms of what Ubiquinol can do in cardiovascular health management."

"I started taking 200 mg of Ubiquinol every day during a very stressful time in my life. My daughter was graduating from high school, my son needed homeschooling and I was having difficulties sleeping. I noticed that Ubiquinol was helping me to function at a high rate and to gain clarity of thought while under stress. In addition, I noticed an increase in energy while taking Ubiquinol. I am thrilled with my results, and plan to continue using Ubiquinol."

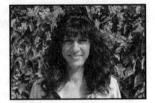

Mary K.
Wilmington, CA

COQ10 DEMYSTIFIED

In a world of familiar vitamins, minerals and herbs, many find Coenzyme Q10 to be enigmatic. Oftentimes, it is only through the word-of-mouth efforts of natural health advocates that people hear the "buzz" about CoQ10. But what exactly is CoQ10?

Simply put, CoQ10 is a fat-soluble, vitamin-like substance that performs tasks that are essential to life itself. In a process called *biosynthesis*, CoQ10 is manufactured by most cells in the body. It circulates widely, is present in all body tissues, and is especially concentrated in organs and tissues that require the most energy.

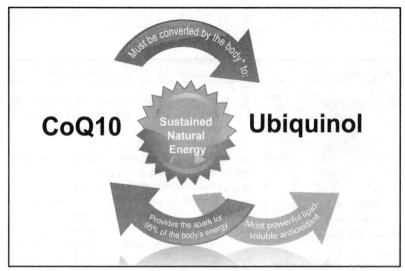

Must be converted by the body* to:

CoQ10

Sustained
Natural
Energy

Ubiquinol

Provides the spark for 95% of the body's energy

Most powerful lipid-soluble antioxidant

*The conversion of CoQ10 to Ubiquinol diminishes with age or oxidative stress

This ubiquitous supernutrient has two main forms: ubiquinone (the "CoQ10" that most know) and Ubiquinol. CoQ10 and Ubiquinol go hand in hand in the body, as partners in a dance known as the "Redox." Redox stands for "reduction" and "oxidation," terms referring to the gain and loss of electrons, respectively. The Ubiquinol form is "reduced;" it has gained extra electrons. When Ubiquinol donates its extra electrons, it "oxidizes" and transforms into CoQ10 (ubiquinone). When CoQ10 is able to gain more extra electrons, it becomes Ubiquinol once again.

And so it goes: As the supernutrient cycles between its two main forms, it is able to perform its critically important, health-promoting, life-sustaining duties: **"sparking" the body's cellular energy and providing powerful antioxidant protection**.

To explain its fundamental role simply: **CoQ10 moves electrons.**[4] While this task may sound trivial, it is, in fact, incredibly profound. At an atomic level, CoQ10 shuttles electrons about – not just in the human body, but throughout most all of Nature's life forms. *CoQ10 is essential for generating life energy.*[5] As CoQ10 moves electrons, it enables life-sustaining chemical reactions in the body beyond liberating energy from food – including neutralizing damaging free radicals and regenerating protective antioxidants. When these chemical reactions are firing on all cylinders, whole-body health thrives.

ANTIOXIDANT IMPORTANCE

Energy's importance is self-evident, but free radicals and antioxidants require some explanation. Free radicals are unstable molecules, an "exhaust" that is produced when the body burns oxygen for energy. External factors like smoking, UV rays, toxins and pollution can also generate free radicals. In a state known as oxidative stress, these out-of-control free radicals smash against cells until they successfully "steal" an electron and gain stability. Free radicals' smashing action is believed to damage cells, DNA and tissues, thereby contributing to aging and age-related diseases.

Antioxidants are valuable because they freely donate electrons to free radicals, stabilizing them and ending their cellular rampage. **Ubiquinol is the most powerful fat-soluble antioxidant that the body produces.** Recall that Ubiquinol is considered the "reduced" form of CoQ10 because it has extra electrons. These extra electrons make Ubiquinol a "charitable" antioxidant substance.

When angry free radicals are trashing the body's cells, friendly **Ubiquinol** donates an extra electron to them. This makes free radicals content and ends their cellular smashing. Vitamin E similarly quenches free radicals, but donating electrons knocks out its power. **Ubiquinol** donates electrons to "spent" vitamin E, "recharging" it so it can continue neutralizing free radical damage. **Ubiquinol** recharges vitamin C the same way.

WHERE DOES COQ10 COME FROM?

Though we can create our own CoQ10, this ability starts to decline around age 20 and enters a tailspin by age 40.[6] With an average life expectancy of nearly 80 years,[7] today our lifespans extend far beyond our CoQ10 biosynthesis ability. Complicating matters further, what little CoQ10 those aged 40+ can muster up through biosynthesis and diet loses power as we age – because as we get older, we also lose the ability to convert CoQ10 into its active form, Ubiquinol.[8]

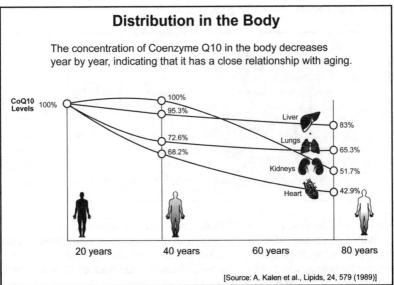

Distribution in the Body

The concentration of Coenzyme Q10 in the body decreases year by year, indicating that it has a close relationship with aging.

CoQ10 Levels 100%

100%
95.3%

Liver 83%

72.6%
68.2%

Lungs 65.3%

Kidneys 51.7%

Heart 42.9%

20 years   40 years   60 years   80 years

[Source: A. Kalen et al., Lipids, 24, 579 (1989)]

In addition to this apparent age-related decline, the following external factors may also play a part in CoQ10 depletion:

- **Missing nutrition**. In order to create CoQ10, the body requires nutritional raw materials including vitamins B2, B6, B12, C, folic acid, niacinamide, pantothenic acid and many trace elements.[9] As nutrient-deficient foods overwhelm the Standard American Diet, it can become increasingly difficult for some to get the nutrition that enables CoQ10 biosynthesis.

- **Statin drugs deplete CoQ10**.[10] Many Americans have turned to statin drugs to manage heart disease – but these statin drugs have been found to deplete CoQ10 levels in the body. Some experts feel that this statin-induced depletion may influence side effects, which may thereby change how well patients follow their statin drug directions.

- **Our Toxic World.** So many free radicals are generated today that much of our CoQ10 stores can be expended "mopping up" these marauding molecules – increasing our need for CoQ10. Oxidative stress also diminishes the body's ability to convert CoQ10 into active Ubiquinol.

Given CoQ10's critical role as an energizing antioxidant, losing our ability to synthesize CoQ10 and convert it to Ubiquinol can lead to dire consequences for health, vitality and overall well-being.

Think of CoQ10 and Ubiquinol as a "dimmer switch" on our vitality. When maxed out with these supernutrients, we glow brightly with health and natural energy. But as aging and environment turn down our CoQ10 and Ubiquinol levels, that healthy, energetic glow fades.

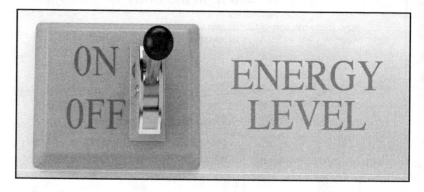

In his book *The Coenzyme Q10 Phenomenon*, Dr. Stephen Sinatra explains, "When a deficiency of Coenzyme Q10 exists, the cellular 'engines' misfire and, over time, they may eventually fail or even die. In essence, without adequate energy the cells would be inefficient, lackluster and vulnerable to free radical attack and disease."[11]

Since free radicals are associated with the premature aging of cells, this CoQ10 deficiency-induced weakening of cellular energy could contribute to a vicious cycle that threatens to sap cellular energy while accelerating aging.

Aging is associated with declining CoQ10 and Ubiquinol levels, which means less cellular energy and less protection against free radicals. As free radical damage increases, aging accelerates – and the cycle continues.

When people learn of the many factors that deplete CoQ10 and Ubiquinol, along with the significant whole-body ramifications this depletion can cause, they naturally want to replenish CoQ10 and Ubiquinol in their bodies. But what is the most effective way to restore these supernutrients for exhilarating health and well-being?

GETTING COQ10

Barring the miraculous discovery of a Fountain of Youth that restores us to our peak CoQ10 biosynthesis years, there are two ways to increase CoQ10 levels in the body: diet or supplementation.

If you radically change your diet to include an abundance of the following foods, you will increase your CoQ10 intake:[12,13]

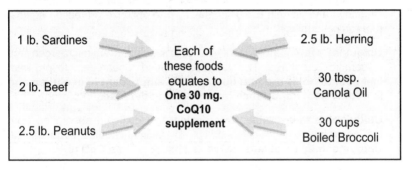

The CoQ10 diet is daunting indeed. Even if you consume these foods in large quantities, your body will still need to convert that dietary CoQ10 into Ubiquinol. Dietary sources are also tricky because CoQ10 is a fragile nutrient; frying foods, for example, reduces CoQ10 level from being marginal to practically nonexistent.

Thankfully, modern science has developed a way to get CoQ10 without having to eat a bucket of sardines. High-quality supplements now deliver CoQ10's supernutrition in two health-promoting forms.

COQ10 CLASSIC: UBIQUINONE

When you take a regular CoQ10 supplement or consume CoQ10-rich foods, you're getting CoQ10's raw form: ubiquinone. If you are under age 40, healthy, and free of undue environmental toxins and stressors, then this form is probably just right for you. At a young age, you will be able to convert CoQ10 into Ubiquinol, enabling full realization of its health benefits.

BREAKTHROUGH SUPPLEMENT: UBIQUINOL

Ubiquinol is the active antioxidant form of CoQ10. When CoQ10 is converted to Ubiquinol, it takes on a dynamic new identity that is responsible for CoQ10's most powerful benefits. Ubiquinol is Superman to CoQ10's Clark Kent, offering powerful supernutrient performance:

- **Ubiquinol** accounts for **over 80%** of the CoQ10 in the plasma of healthy young individuals, drawing a link between Ubiquinol and youthful exuberance.

- **Ubiquinol** provides the **spark** for most of the body's energy production.[14]

- **Ubiquinol** plays a vital role in generating energy to power organs such as the heart, kidneys, liver and lungs.

- **Ubiquinol** is considered the strongest lipid-soluble antioxidant that is synthesized. Because it is lipid-soluble, Ubiquinol may protect cell membranes, proteins, and our very own DNA.[15]

- **Ubiquinol** "regenerates" other antioxidants, including standbys like vitamin C and vitamin E.[16] This may help to optimize protection against free radical damage.

- **Ubiquinol** is a vital component of all cells in nature, from microorganisms to complex creatures. This fact has inspired researchers to proclaim that **"Ubiquinol is the first lipid-soluble antioxidant in evolution and is of universal importance for antioxidant defenses in biology."**[17]

- **Ubiquinol** is bioavailable; it has exhibited significant absorption from the gastrointestinal tract.[18] Additionally, animal studies suggest that **Ubiquinol may be at least twice as absorbable as CoQ10.**[19]

Ubiquinol as a supplement is appealing because it is "ready-to-use" by the body, so there's no lag or energy lost in the conversion process. Highly absorbable, Ubiquinol is simply easier for those aged 40+ to use.

NUTRITIONAL INNOVATION

Though scientists have been aware of CoQ10 and Ubiquinol for decades, Ubiquinol proved to be an extremely fragile nutrient that converts back to CoQ10 as soon as it touches oxygen. Because of its seemingly limitless health-enhancing potential, Ubiquinol's challenges did not faze researchers – it became a "Holy Grail" to nutritional supplement manufacturers.

After 10 years of research, the secret to producing a safe and stable supplement form of Ubiquinol was discovered. KANEKA QH™ Ubiquinol represents the first bio-identical Ubiquinol in supplement form. KANEKA QH™ is now available in over 50 nutritional supplement formulations.

KANEKA QH™'s emergence at this point in history is uncanny. In 2005, there were 78.2 million baby boomers.[20] In 2006, 8,000 people turned 60 each day.[21] Today, the demographic that is unable to efficiently convert CoQ10 to Ubiquinol has a new way to obtain Ubiquinol's significant health benefits – just when they may need it the most.

Did you know?
CoQ10 contains *potential* antioxidant activity, but first the body must convert it into Ubiquinol. Supplemental Ubiquinol requires no conversion and therefore is immediately ready for the body to use. For peak antioxidant benefits, remember: only the Ubiquinol form of CoQ10 is an active antioxidant.

DAWNING RESEARCH

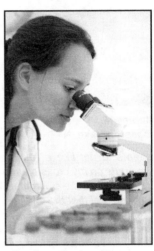

Since Ubiquinol is a nutritional supplement newcomer, clinical trials are still in early phases. One groundbreaking early Ubiquinol study, however, has been completed. In this new study, seven patients with advanced congestive heart failure who were struggling to absorb supplemental CoQ10 were switched over from CoQ10 to equivalent levels of Ubiquinol (ranging 450 - 600 mg per day). After the switch, patients' CoQ10 blood levels increased from an average of 1.6 micrograms/mL to an average of 6.5, while ejection fraction – a measure of how well the heart is pumping blood – improved from an average of 22% to an average of 39% (ejection fraction below 35% is considered a life-threatening crisis). These changes led researchers to conclude that Ubiquinol has dramatically improved absorption in patients with severe heart failure, and is accompanied by an increase in CoQ10 plasma levels that is associated with clinical improvement. The researchers suggest that earlier Ubiquinol administration might have an even greater benefit, and that more clinical trials of Ubiquinol are "anxiously awaited."[18]

COQ10 VS. UBIQUINOL

For the sake of simplicity, this book will refer primarily to CoQ10, as this is the form that is most familiar. But as you read on, consider which CoQ10 form might be best suited for you. Some evidence suggests that if you are over 40, taking statin drugs, or you believe you might be suffering from oxidative stress associated with our toxic, free radical-laden world, then pre-converted, ready-to-use **Ubiquinol** may be better for you.

Let's read on to discover how the supernutrition of CoQ10 and Ubiquinol may translate to significant gains in health and well being.

Bioenergetic Nutrition

"I have committed to CoQ10 primarily because of its role as a formidable weapon in promoting a healthy heart. I was only 15 when my dad died of a heart attack at age 46. Right then and there I decided to do whatever was necessary to stave off this killer that has also claimed two of dad's brothers before their time. For the last 40 years I have enthusiastically pursued a lifestyle focused on optimal nutrition, regular exercise, and targeted daily supplementation.

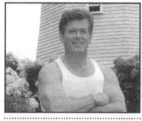

CoQ10 became part of my regimen in 1998 and remains an essential component in the daily battle to stave off the effects of stress and the natural aging process.

Truthfully, I have been quite surprised at the surge in energy during my weight training! My reps increased and my stamina has improved markedly. I am still cranking out curls and presses at an energy level that defies my 59 years! This is great, since after age 40 a natural metabolic slow-down takes a toll on us all, and CoQ10

James M.
Ballston Lake, NY

seems to act like a rejuvenating supercharger. I power through aerobic workouts on my cross-country ski machine with greater intensity and duration. This supports the claim that CoQ10 optimizes the energy value of my food.

I also feel that the immune system boost provided by CoQ10 helped me to a speedy recovery after my total knee replacement surgery in 2006. But my sense of well-being is the real charmer here! Knowing that I can rely on the purity and efficacy of this supplement is a real confidence-booster. I now enjoy a fuller life thanks to the restorative power unleashed by CoQ10. I heartily beckon everyone to jump on board the 'CoQ10 EXPRESS!'"

"At age 53, my health was failing. My energy levels had dropped so low that I was unable to continue my favorite hobby: tinkering in my wood and metal shop. My cardiologist, Dr. Langsjoen, put me on Ubiquinol. After taking it and following other prescribed health regimens, my doctor told me my CoQ10 plasma levels had almost doubled. With increased energy levels, I began to feel strong enough to start tinkering in my workshop again – and was cleared by my doctor to celebrate my golden wedding anniversary onboard a cruise ship. I had never even heard of Ubiquinol, but after seeing the results and how it makes me feel – I'm a believer!"

Joe M.
Tyler, TX

One of the key markers of a life well-lived is energy. When both body and mind are energized, life is loaded with possibilities – traveling, socializing and engaging in any number of recreational activities are all easily accessible when energy levels are high.

Energy also equates to health, allowing for invigorated exercise, a motivated attitude, a robust disposition and an overall enjoyment of life. After all, in any person's life, no major memorable achievements are accomplished on low energy. *Life-enhancing energy simply wouldn't be possible without CoQ10 and Ubiquinol.*

CELLULAR BIOENERGETICS

While it may sound like terminology from a Hollywood sci-fi movie, cellular bioenergetics is the process in which energy flows and is exchanged through living things. It is a crucial component of biochemistry, and this "chemical bond energy," a groundbreaking 1981 study indicates, "is the exclusive source of utilizable energy in biological systems."[22] **CoQ10 is essential for the bioenergetic process**, since it plays a crucial role in the creation of cellular energy in the mitochondria, which serve as microscopic power plants in every cell of the body.

Did you know?
Eighty percent of the body's CoQ10 and Ubiquinol located in our cells can be found in the mitochondria.[23]

If the body is properly supplied with CoQ10, mitochondria are primed to operate at a highly efficient pace because they are supercharged with the fuel they need to generate energy. Without CoQ10, mitochondria can't produce energy, leading to a chain reaction that echoes throughout the body. Lacking fuel, trillions of cells can become sluggish, an adverse effect that resonates in every aspect of day-to-day human function.

CoQ10 and Ubiquinol supplements literally provide a boost to the system, supporting energy production in practically every single cell. This surge of cellular reinforcements may bolster body and mind by promoting and sustaining natural energy.

Did you know?
CoQ10 is abundant in the organs and systems that use the most energy: the heart, liver, kidneys, pancreas, brain, and immune system. In fact, CoQ10 is most concentrated in the heart, making the nutrient particularly important for heart health.[24]

Many people report an increase in life energy after they begin CoQ10 supplementation. Studies have validated these testimonials, suggesting that supplemental CoQ10 may help to fight fatigue and supercharge vitality:

- A 2008 study investigated CoQ10's impact on fatigue. The researchers discovered that healthy subjects performing bicycle trials who were given 300 mg of CoQ10 were considerably less fatigued than their placebo-taking peers. In addition, researchers reported that the CoQ10 group rated higher on physical performance and had a quicker recovery time.[25]

- In another study, researchers reported that both athletically trained and untrained participants who were taking CoQ10 appeared to enjoy better exercise performance. Researchers said that consistent, ongoing CoQ10 supplementation also appeared to extend the amount of time people could exercise before they reached exhaustion. Additionally, researchers found that those taking CoQ10 only one time still had a higher muscle concentration of CoQ10 and experienced less oxidative stress before and during exercise.[26]

Studies like these suggest that CoQ10 and Ubiquinol may be helpful supplements for both athletes and casual weekend warriors – because they may energize the body, extend exertion time, reduce recovery time and neutralize the damaging free radicals that are generated during exercise.[27]

POWER GENERATOR

On a very basic level, CoQ10 sustains natural energy, allowing the bioenergetics process to work its molecular magic. This, in turn, supports energy production further by utilizing ubiquinone to aid impaired mitochondria. CoQ10 is required for energy production in cells, helping them to use the oxygen they receive and maintain mitochondrial membranes and cellular membrane fluidity.[28]

CoQ10 plays a vital role in the production of adenosine triphosphate (ATP), a nucleotide that stores energy in the cell, by assisting in converting carbohydrates and fats into ATP, which then moves chemical energy within cells as a part of the greater metabolic process.[29] Although CoQ10's role in generating energy is complex, it boils down to CoQ10 molecules helping other enzymes by shuttling protons and electrons, acting as a "courier" whose absence would mean a complete energy generation failure.

ENERGY IS LIFE

CoQ10 provides integral assistance in creating and maintaining the natural energy that is so closely tied to health, longevity, happiness and quality of life. In addition to the overarching impact of dynamic energy that we feel in our day-to-day lives, CoQ10 and Ubiquinol enable processes in the body that we can't always feel – such as the functioning of our vital organs and body systems. Read on to learn about how CoQ10's energizing ability helps power our organs to peak healthy performance.

Lifelong Heart Health Support

"CoQ10 has helped my patients and my practice immeasurably."

"I recommend CoQ10 to all of my adult patients. To me, it is a 'desert island supplement;' I would not want to ever be without it. CoQ10 is always in my top five supplements. The reasons for that are several fold but the most

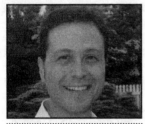

Fred Pescatore, MD, MPH, CCN
Author, *The Hamptons Diet*
Co-Host, *New Vitality Live*

compelling is that CoQ10 is so well clinically researched and documented to have positive effects in supporting the cardiovascular system. CoQ10 also offers cholesterol support and acts as a super antioxidant – which means it helps other antioxidants do their job more efficiently. CoQ10 is found in every cell in our body and helps our mitochondria to function at the level they are supposed to. Therefore, how can it not help our cells and our health? I can honestly say that Coenzyme Q10 has helped my patients and my practice immeasurably.

"I am thrilled with the results..."

"After a blood test, my physician recommended that I begin taking CoQ10. At the time my HDL [good cholesterol] was 76.0 and LDL [bad cholesterol] was 127. Now, less than one year later, my HDL is 77.8 and my LDL is 108. I am pleased to report that the addition of CoQ10 has made a definite improvement to my cholesterol levels. I am thrilled with the results and have started my husband on this supplement.

My husband is 78 years young and I will be 76 in less than two months. We have a regimen of supplements that I have put together following a great deal of study over the past 15 years. Yoga has also been an important part of my staying young program; I do an hour and a half daily and have added Pilates to my routine. In addition, I walk each day for 20 minutes.

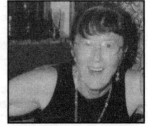

My only wish is that more folks our age could be made aware of the importance of supplementation and exercise!"

Ethel J. Benson, AZ

CoQ10's energy-promoting activity is especially crucial in the body's hardest-working organ: the heart. Every day, the heart beats 100,000 times and pumps 1,800 gallons of blood. Clearly, the heart requires a tremendous amount of energy to achieve peak performance. Heart problems have multiple causes, but heart failure is always characterized by energy depletion.[30]

Heart disease is the #1 killer in America, responsible for nearly 700,000 deaths each year – that's approximately 29% of all deaths.[31] CoQ10 deficiency may be one of the reasons behind the heart disease epidemic: **Research has consistently shown that cardiac patients have diminished CoQ10 levels in their hearts,** and that patients with the worst heart disease have the lowest CoQ10 levels.

Researchers have proclaimed that for those with heart problems, CoQ10 therapy can result in "a profound increase both in cardiac function and quality of life."[32] Studies suggest that CoQ10 and Ubiquinol may help to promote heart health by performing a diversity of cardioprotective actions:

- **Promoting and maintaining peak cardiac energy.**[33] Cardiac energy depletion is frequently found in heart failure patients.

- **Protecting the heart tissues from free radical damage.** This protection may extend to the fragile DNA of the heart's energy-producing mitochondria cells.

- **Inhibiting the oxidation of LDL ("bad") cholesterol.**[34] Oxidized LDL is associated with clogged, unhealthy arteries.

- **Reducing blood cell size and stabilizing cell membranes,** helping to reduce the risk of blood clot formation.[35]

- **Helping the heart beat with greater output, stability and efficiency.** This benefit may help cardiomyopathy, in which the heart weakens and pumps less blood.[36]

- **Maintaining blood pressure that's already in a normal range.** High blood pressure increases risk for stroke and heart attack.

These potential benefits all point to a stronger, healthier, more energetic, better-functioning heart. This is why *CoQ10 is most studied for its impact on heart health.*

Mother Nature gifted us the ability to synthesize, convert and utilize CoQ10 in order to energize and protect our very cells. Further, Nature's wisdom concentrated CoQ10 in the heart, where this energizing protection helps keep us alive.

But when CoQ10 begins to disappear from the heart, cardiovascular health problems appear to manifest. And disturbingly, in the face of a heart disease epidemic, an ironic twist of Western Medicine appears to be hurting our hearts just as it tries to help them – by depleting CoQ10 just when we need it more than ever.

THE STATIN PARADOX

HMG-CoA reductase inhibitors (statins) are drugs that are used to treat heart disease, especially high cholesterol. As heart disease skyrockets, statins have become the most commonly prescribed drugs in America.[37] In 2003-2004, 23 million Americans took statins, including 27% of adults over age 65.[38]

While statin drugs help many Americans' heart health, they present a paradoxical side effect: **statin drugs deplete CoQ10 levels in the body**, which may leave the heart susceptible to a number of different negative health conditions.

The good news is that experts have proclaimed that CoQ10 deficiency that is caused by statins **can be completely reversed with CoQ10 supplementation**[39] – thus restoring heart health-promoting energy and antioxidant protection. Although a petition has been filed with the FDA requesting that statin drug labels include a CoQ10 recommendation, the petition remains unrealized.[40] Until such labeling becomes law, many are taking statin matters into their own hands by taking CoQ10 into their hearts.

"I am 87 years old and in excellent health. For many years I have tended towards high cholesterol. My doctor prescribed a statin drug. This was about 15 years ago and my energy and optimism were low. I read several books by leading health authorities and doctors and one statement showed up repeatedly: CoQ10 is depleted due to age and statin drugs. I began taking 50 mg of CoQ10; I have recently increased to 100 mg daily.

I am proud to say that two years ago, I felt optimistic and energetic enough to make a big life change with my daughter, moving from Florida to Texas. I now attend yoga, power walking and strength training classes four days a week. I am active in church, family and cultural events, and am completing a manuscript of my life story.

In addition, my regular checkups (heart, blood pressure, etc.) are normal. I attribute my wellness in large part to CoQ10, which aids in keeping all my systems functioning. I have convinced my 53-year-old daughter of the importance of CoQ10 and her energy level has greatly improved since she began taking it."

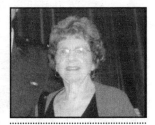

Mary S.
Farmers Branch, TX

Heart disease is a catchall phrase that refers to a number of different conditions. Chronic heart failure, for example, is a universal term referring to the heart's inability to pump enough blood – but this state can have several contributing factors such as cardiomyopathy (weakening of the heart), high blood pressure, atherosclerosis (clogged, hardened arteries), diabetes and others. Studies suggest that as CoQ10 promotes cardiac energy and helps fight free radical damage, it can deliver multifaceted heart health benefits:

- In the Italian Multicenter Study, the largest CoQ10 study to date, over 1,100 heart failure patients were given 50 to 150 mg of CoQ10 daily for three months. At study's end, cardiologists reported that even though the trial was relatively brief, **80% of the patients enjoyed positive results by taking CoQ10** as a complementary therapy. Improvement rates among specific heart failure symptoms were recorded as follows: edema, 76.9%; arrhythmia 62%; palpitations 75.7%; and pulmonary rales 78.4%. Overall, 54% of the subjects enjoyed improvement in three or more heart failure symptoms; researchers suggested this could be interpreted as an enhancement in quality of life.[41]

- Another analysis suggested that CoQ10 promotes heart health even when taken at a lower level for a shorter time span. In the study, 1,715 chronic heart failure patients were given 50 mg CoQ10 daily for four weeks while still receiving conventional therapy. The study authors reported that CoQ10, in conjunction with conventional treatment, was associated with statistically significant improvement; in some cases, this improvement was observed in as little as two weeks. Physicians' assessment of the patients was also positive, **with 86.5% reporting "fairly good" to "excellent" CoQ10 therapy results.**[42]

CoQ10's heart therapy efficacy as assessed by 378 physicians:

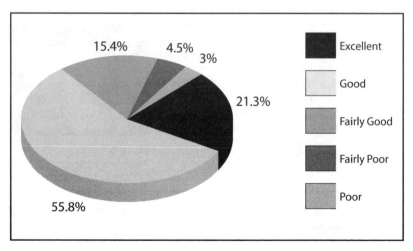

- The New York Heart Association (NYHA) Functional Classification is a rating system that conveys the extent of heart failure. The system rates cardiovascular patients from I (no daily limitations) to IV (significant limitations, confined to bedrest). One study evaluated 424 cardiovascular patients' response to CoQ10 therapy (in addition to conventional therapy) according to the NYHA scale. Patients took an average of 242 mg of CoQ10 per day, and were tracked for an average of 17.8 months. At study's end, researchers reported that 87.2% of the cardiovascular patients taking supplemental COQ10 enjoyed an improvement; 58% improved by one NYHA class, 28% by two NYHA classes, and 1.2% by three NYHA classes.[43]

The evidence supporting CoQ10 and Ubiquinol as heart health champions gets even more compelling. Additional studies have hinted at expansive cardiovascular health-promoting benefits.

BAD CHOLESTEROL
As it turns out, LDL cholesterol – "bad cholesterol" – gets even worse when it is "oxidized" by free radicals. Oxidized LDL is strongly associated with risk for heart disease and atherosclerosis (clogged, hardened arteries).[44] Research has shown that taking CoQ10 as a supplement results in greater concentrations of Ubiquinol being carried in the bloodstream on LDL cholesterol.[45] Here, Ubiquinol's antioxidant power appears to support arterial health by helping to inhibit LDL cholesterol from being oxidized and regenerating vitamin E for even more antioxidant protection.[46]

BLOOD PRESSURE
73 million Americans aged 20+ have high blood pressure (hypertension), all of whom face elevated risk for strokes, heart attacks, heart failure,

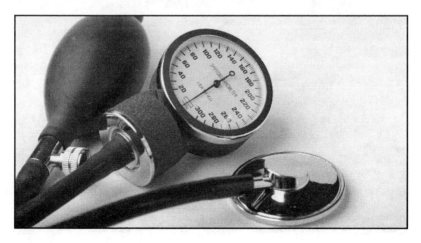

kidney problems and aneurysm.[47] A recent meta-analysis broke down the results of 12 clinical trials totaling 362 hypertension patients. Overall, researchers found that those who underwent CoQ10 therapy enjoyed blood pressure reductions. The researchers concluded that CoQ10 "has the potential in hypertensive patients to lower systolic blood pressure by up to 17 mm Hg and diastolic blood pressure by up to 10 mm Hg." CoQ10 is known to help maintain blood pressure that is already in a normal range.[48]

Did you know?
In Japan, CoQ10 is "prescribed" as an adjunct to standard therapy to patients with failing hearts, and has been approved as a heart disease treatment since 1974 – representing the first commercial application of CoQ10. Today, over 250 different preparations containing CoQ10 are available in Japan to treat heart conditions.[49]

ISCHEMIA & ANGINA

In a condition called ischemia, blood flow to the heart is reduced, which can lead to painful angina episodes. Poor blood flow to the heart can be caused by blood clots, clogged arteries, rapid heartbeat, strokes and other causes. When ischemia is corrected, the resulting rush of blood to the heart can flood it with oxygen – paradoxically, generating tremendous oxidative stress on the heart.[50] Ubiquinol's antioxidant power may quench these free radicals and protect the heart, which is part of the reason why leading researchers have suggested that CoQ10 may be a safe, promising way to alleviate angina pectoris. Researchers have revealed that angina patients taking 150 mg per day of CoQ10 are better able to exert themselves without experiencing chest discomfort.[51]

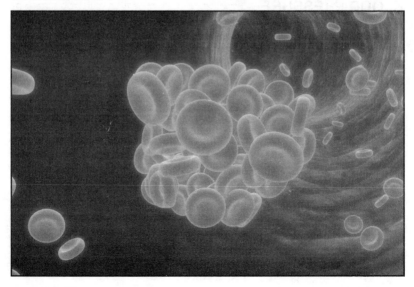

HEART SURGERY

Proactive, preventive health strategies are always better than waiting to treat sickness with reactive medicine. But even the most diligent preventive heart health strategies can still fall short, leaving surgery as the only option. Some evidence suggests that CoQ10, in addition to promoting and maintaining heart health, may help those who are both preparing for and recovering from heart surgery:[52]

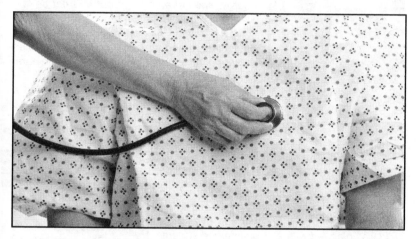

- Twenty high-risk patients with CoQ10 deficiency were selected for CoQ10 treatment prior to bypass surgery or bypass with valve replacement surgery. Patients received 100 mg per day of CoQ10 for 14 days before surgery and 30 days after surgery. Prior to surgery, the supplementation increased CoQ10 levels in the heart tissue and blood; heart tissue energy also received a boost. After surgery, CoQ10 was preserved in blood and heart tissues in the treatment group. Researchers concluded that **cardiac pumping and left ventricle ejection fraction were significantly improved in the CoQ10 group. Additionally, the CoQ10 group had an accelerated recovery of three to five days,** compared to the 15-30 day recovery period of the control group. Researchers concluded that the results suggest CoQ10 may preserve the heart muscle during heart surgery, and that a positive relationship can be drawn between CoQ10 levels, heart energy, cardiac function and postoperative recovery time.[53]

All of this evidence combines to reveal a profound nutritional truth that holds the potential to both improve the quality and quantity of our years:

CoQ10 supports the arterial and cardiovascular systems –
helping to promote *and* maintain a healthy heart!

Whole-Life Vitality

"The results have been amazing..."

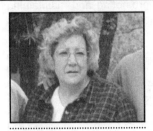

Betty M.
St. Paul, MN

I would recommend that everyone take CoQ10. I have felt so much better, have great energy, and I'm able to go out and not be laid up all the time with health problems.

My grandson has tinnitus from loud work equipment. I read an article on how CoQ10, as a superior antioxidant, helps ringing in the ears. My grandson has been taking 100 mg daily for the past two months now and has noticed a positive difference already. I'll be taking CoQ10 as a daily benefit for my health... it's great!"

"My energy is boundless..."

"CoQ10 has made such an improvement in my health, I was bursting at the seams to let you know! I was born in 1938 and even as a child was plagued with a weak immune system. My children are amazed – they can't believe that a capsule can change your whole life. I just ordered several bottles to distribute among them, especially now that the cold and flu season is upon us.

Three years ago, before CoQ10, I was a tired, weak woman. I read about CoQ10 and now my energy is boundless and my life is vibrant at 70 years of age."

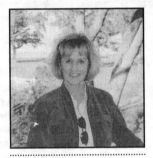

Murlene N.
Jackson, MS

What do periodontitis, migraines, immunity, tinnitus and reproductive problems all have in common? More often than not, these afflictions are associated with low CoQ10 levels. Already well-established in the areas of heart health, energy and antioxidant activity, science is now exploding with even more exciting CoQ10 and Ubiquinol health benefits. In fact, it is becoming increasingly clear to experts that CoQ10 and Ubiquinol may offer comprehensive health benefits including applications for cognitive function, migraines, inflammatory response and more.

SMILING FOR NO REASON: GUM HEALTH

Sure, we all brush our teeth and try to floss daily. But for many of us, this routine is not enough. Gum disease is often genetic, afflicting many for no other reason than the fact that it runs in the family. Up to a third of the population may have inherited a predisposition to gum problems like periodontitis, the dreaded gum disease that destroys the soft tissue and bone supporting teeth, potentially leading to tooth loss. Luckily, promising research is now suggesting that CoQ10 may help to support gum health.

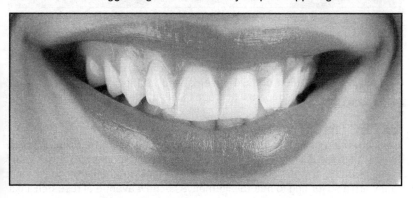

- One study investigating the link between a deficiency of Coenzyme Q10 and periodontal disease found startling results: about 60% of the 40 diseased gingival tissues showed a deficiency of CoQ10.[54] In other findings, CoQ10 applied to pockets of diseased gum tissue appeared to significantly reduce infection.[55]

"I am a faithful user of CoQ10. In 1990 I had bleeding gums and a history of soft gums. I lost many teeth as a child. I found a book entitled 'The Miracle of Antioxidant CoQ10.' This book clarified how this coenzyme works and explained that the Western diet is deficient in CoQ10. I am 73 years old, have been taking CoQ10 since 1990, and still have some of my own teeth. In addition, my M.D. tells me that I have the blood pressure of a 20-year-old."

**Patricia G.
Ashland, OR**

NATURAL MIGRAINE CARE

Because a large amount of people who suffer from these debilitating, agonizing and often frequent migraine headaches do not respond to pharmacological interventions, many are seeking alternative remedies. Promising preliminary evidence suggests that Coenzyme Q10 may help:

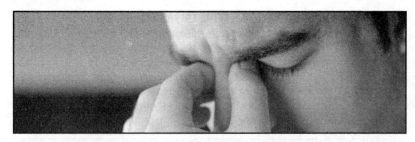

- One stand-out study suggests that at a level of 150 mg of CoQ10 per day, 61.3% of patients studied had a greater than 50% reduction in amount of days with a migraine.[56] In another study, authors reported finding CoQ10 deficiency in children who suffer from migraine headaches. In fact, a large portion of child patients who had low CoQ10 levels were found to have a third below average levels of the important nutrient.[57]

EXPECTING THE BEST

Science is increasingly conscious of the link between CoQ10 and reproductive health. With the $3 billion fertility industry amassing more profit every year, many couples are still struggling to achieve their reproductive goals, and many are also turning to natural alternatives. A new avenue of research links CoQ10 to male fertility, specifically with the condition of idiopathic asthenozoospermia, or low sperm motility.

- Experts suggest that CoQ10 might improve sperm fertilization rates, sperm count and sperm motility. Researchers theorize that we are exposed to environmental toxins which accumulate in the body as we age; CoQ10 helps provide proper antioxidant defenses that may protect sperm cells from such attacks.[58]

MUSIC TO YOUR EARS

What can range from a nuisance for some to a life-altering condition for others, tinnitus (ringing in the ears) distresses an estimated 12 million people in the United States alone. Chronic tinnitus can interfere with the body's natural means to maintain well-being, such as ability to relax, sleep

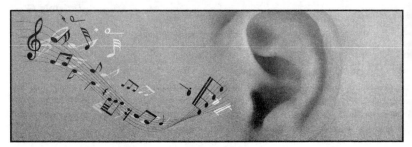

and concentrate. Tinnitus sufferers may look to CoQ10 supplementation as a natural way to help themselves:

- In one study, German doctors administered 100 mg of CoQ10 to 20 tinnitus patients three times daily. At the 12-week study's completion, researchers concluded that patients taking CoQ10 had reduced tinnitus by 36 percent.[59]

IMMUNE BOOSTER, INFECTION WARRIOR

Perhaps some of the most exciting developments in CoQ10 health are its applications for immunity. While vitamin and nutritional deficiencies have been long associated with immuno-deficiencies, researchers believe that CoQ10 is also a vital component for the peak immune system function. During a 1981 conference on Coenzyme Q10, researchers:

1. Established the role of CoQ10 as an effective immunomodulating agent.

2. Established that aging and disease both create a CoQ10 deficiency.

3. Surmised that CoQ10, at the mitochondrial level, is vital for optimal immune function.

4. Found that, due to its lack of toxicity, CoQ10 is an ideal candidate for clinical application in cases where immunity is not at favorable levels.

5. Concluded that infections and immunity-related "diseases of aging" should be treated as "diseases of bioenergetics."

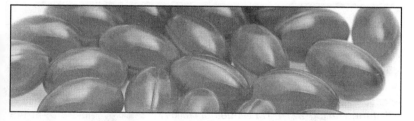

Scientists have asserted that CoQ10's powerful support appears to modulate the body's immune system functioning, thereby neutralizing inflammatory pathogens.[60]

THE WONDER NUTRIENT!

CoQ10 deficiency appears to be the common denominator behind a broad spectrum of conditions. Even as you are reading this, science is continuing to investigate and discern intriguing new applications for two of the most exciting, far-reaching supplements available today: CoQ10 and its active form, Ubiquinol.

Young at Heart

"I look and feel much younger!"

"On October 28, 1991, I was on the highway going 60 miles an hour when a drunk driver going 80 miles an hour hit me. My car turned over twice. I immediately went into a coma. The Jaws of Life had to cut off the roof of my car to get me out. An ambulance took me to the hospital. After five weeks

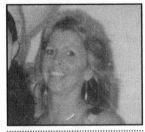

Shari D.
Middleburg Heights, OH

they moved me to New Medico in West Palm Beach, where they taught me to walk, talk and other functions.

After five months, my sister and I flew from Florida to my new home in Ohio with my mother and stepfather. After reading about many vitamins and herbs, I started taking CoQ10. Within a month, I had enough energy to join a health club, which I go to for two to three hours, three days a week. CoQ10 gave me so much energy, I also became a volunteer at a local Health Center.

I have now been working out and volunteering for 10 years, and I still love doing it. I have told all my family and friends about the miracle of CoQ10. I have more than enough energy all day because of CoQ10 – I take one every day. I recently celebrated my 49th birthday, but I look and feel much younger!"

"I have a little extra bounce in my step..."

"Following a stroke at age 47, I realized I needed to proactively improve my health. I started reading labels, closely watching what I ate, and became a huge advocate for the health benefits of antioxidants.

I started taking 100 mg of Ubiquinol per day. Within just a couple of days I started to notice improvements. I felt like I had more energy. I no longer had the urge to snack because I was bored. Now my diet is 95 percent better than it used to be, I am sleeping better at night and

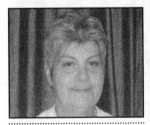

Virginia V.
Fayetteville, NC

I have a little extra bounce in my step each day. My doctor has also seen improvement in my quarterly blood tests since I started supplementing with Ubiquinol.

I am 54 years old and I feel like I am in my early 40s. I truly believe this is due to my taking Ubiquinol. I will definitely continue to take it to improve not only my life, but my lifespan."

From the evidence presented in this book, it's clear that CoQ10 and Ubiquinol are truly remarkable natural, health-promoting substances. Assigned the seemingly simple task of carrying electrons, CoQ10 and Ubiquinol's sub-atomic influence supports health benefits that appear to expand and multiply.

As powerful as the scientific evidence is that validates CoQ10's health-promoting power, the testimonials from real people – your neighbors, friends, or even loved ones – may be the most compelling evidence of all. When taking these supernutrients in supplement form, people report transcendent benefits that elevate them to a state of exhilarating well-being, using phrases such as "miraculous" and "life-changing" as they describe CoQ10's impact. Many even report that they feel younger – as if CoQ10 and Ubiquinol help them defy aging and turn back the clock.

This youthful phenomenon is not just an illusion. In fact, leading researchers have proclaimed that "There is ample evidence that high levels of ubiquinone [CoQ10]… slow the detrimental biochemical, structural and other changes that occur with aging in all mammals."[61]

The Free Radical Theory Of Aging may help explain why CoQ10 is associated with youthful energy. Developed by pioneering aging researcher Dr. Denham Harman in 1954, the theory postulates that those aggressive, unstable free radicals you've been reading about actually accelerate aging by damaging our cells.[62] Under the Free Radical Theory Of Aging, **Ubiquinol** could represent a powerful force in the quest to stay young. After all, not only is Ubiquinol one of the most powerful fat-soluble antioxidants, it recharges other antioxidants to optimize our natural defenses.

Since over 80% of the CoQ10 concentration in the blood of healthy young people is Ubiquinol, it has been suggested that when this antioxidant form of CoQ10 is circulating abundantly, reaching all tissues, we are closer to matching a natural state of youthfulness.

In addition to promoting youthful energy, CoQ10 may help to fight the signs of visible aging – a belief that is exemplified in the dramatic increase of serums, salves, skin-care products and "wrinkle" or "anti-aging" creams that feature CoQ10. These formulations are also rooted in science and backed by research and development. A clinical investigation of topical CoQ10 led researchers to conclude that after six weeks of daily treatment, wrinkle depth was reduced by 27%; after 10 weeks, fine lines and wrinkles were reduced by 43%.[63]

Do you need more reason to consider CoQ10 as a supplement that supports healthy aging? Animal studies have led researchers to suggest that CoQ10, in conjunction with a polyunsaturated fats-rich diet, *may even extend lifespan.*[64]

YOUTH PERSONIFIED

If you found the legendary Fountain of Youth and deeply drank its cool, refreshing waters, how would you feel? Your heart would beat stronger, with renewed vitality. You'd experience an invigorating resurgence of pure, natural energy. Gums would be restored to pristine pink health, immune performance would flourish, and even reproductive health would get a boost. Skin would glow with healthy radiance, becoming soft, smooth and supple. As you have read in this book, scientific evidence suggests that CoQ10 and Ubiquinol may promote these results.

In a healthy, youthful state of nature, we possess the ability to create our own CoQ10 and convert it to its powerful active form, Ubiquinol. But as age and environmental factors trigger an inevitable decline in our ability to create, convert, and utilize CoQ10, energy levels wane and chronic ill-health conditions take root. But just as modern medicine extended our lives beyond our ability to create and convert CoQ10, modern science has now caught up – by developing innovative natural supplements that replenish our CoQ10 and Ubiquinol levels.

The great Irish playwright George Bernard Shaw once said, "Youth is wasted on the young." This may no longer be the case. With CoQ10 supplements, and especially with the breakthrough nutritional support of Ubiquinol supplements, we may be empowered to reclaim and relish youthful exuberance – even as we age.

As you've seen in many of these testimonials, a resurgence of sustained life-energy is just the beginning. Many who supplement with CoQ10 and Ubiquinol suddenly feel motivated to start working out, doing Pilates, performing yoga and playing tennis. As Lucy O. so eloquently stated in the first story in this book, CoQ10 may hold the key to helping people "make their dreams come true."

In maintaining youthful levels of CoQ10 and Ubiquinol through supplementation, we may help to promote the amazing quality of life we enjoyed when we were younger – with healthy, energetic bodies; positive, bright outlooks; and a zest for living that we carry in our hearts every single day.

CHECKLIST

- ☑ Age, environmental stressors, statin drugs and poor health states are all associated with a gradual decline in CoQ10 levels.

- ☑ Additionally, as we age we lose our ability to convert CoQ10 into its active antioxidant form: **Ubiquinol**.

- ☑ CoQ10 supports heart health, artery health, cellular energy, antioxidant defenses and healthy aging. CoQ10 also helps maintain blood pressure that's already in a normal range.

- ☑ CoQ10 and Ubiquinol levels have been shown to be suppressed in individuals with mitochondrial, cardiovascular, neurological, liver-related and diabetes-related conditions.

COQ10

CoQ10 is a fat-soluble, vitamin-like substance found in nearly every cell in the human body. Dietary sources of CoQ10 include organ meats, sardines and spinach. CoQ10 supplements have been available for 30 years. Some CoQ10 supplementation tips:

- Since it is fat-soluble, CoQ10 absorption may be enhanced if CoQ10 is taken with foods that contain fat.[65]

- For young, healthy individuals, CoQ10 should usually be sufficient for supplementation needs. Healthy adults in their 20s and 30s are better able to utilize CoQ10 and convert it into active Ubiquinol. For these people, supplementing with CoQ10 may be the most efficient way to raise CoQ10 levels.

- 30-60 mg/day is recommended to prevent CoQ10 deficiency. It is suggested that servings over 100 mg/day be administered in divided doses.

UBIQUINOL

Ubiquinol is the CoQ10 form that accounts for many of the significant health benefits associated with CoQ10, and is believed to be one of the most powerful fat-soluble antioxidants. Thanks to a nutritional breakthrough, Ubiquinol recently became available in supplement form. Some Ubiquinol supplementation tips:

- For individuals who are 40+, or for those who are affected by chronic disease, Ubiquinol is likely a better supplement choice than CoQ10. In these individuals, the body's ability to produce CoQ10 and convert it into Ubiquinol is diminished.

- Those who are older or suspect they have decreased CoQ10 due to sickness or increased oxidative stress may want to start supplementing with 200-300 mg of Ubiquinol per day for two weeks and then switch to 100 mg per day to maintain Ubiquinol levels.[66]

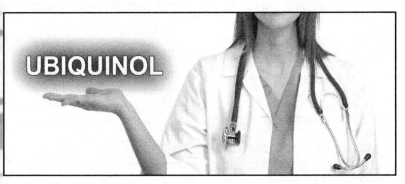

SAFETY NOTES

- Both CoQ10 and Ubiquinol have been shown to be overwhelmingly safe.[67] This should come as no surprise, since they are naturally-occuring substances in the body. Though CoQ10 and Ubiquinol are completely safe, you should always consult with a qualified healthcare practitioner before beginning any nutritional supplement program.

References

1. Ernster L, Dallner G: Biochemical, physiological and medical aspects of ubiquinol function. Biochem Biophys Acta 1271: 195-204, 1995

2. Weber G, Jakobsen TS, Mortensen SA, et al. Antioxidative effect of dietary coenzyme Q10 in human blood plasma. Int J Vitam Nutr Res 1994;64:311-5.

3. Bliznakov EG. Coenzyme Q10, Lipid-Lowering Drugs (Statins) and Cholesterol: A Present Day Pandora's Box. The Journal of the American Nutraceutical Association Vol. 5, No. 3, Summer 2002.

4. Ubiquinol: the Other Half of the CoQ10 Story. Connolly K. Available at: http://www.americanwellnessnetwork.com/index.php/20071204939/Ubiquinol-and-CoQ10.html

5. Goldberg B, Trivieri L, Anderson JW. Alternative Medicine: The Definitive Guide. Published by Celestial Arts, 2002

6. Kalen (1989). Lipids,24,579-584

7. http://www.cdc.gov/nchs/fastats/lifexpec.htm

8. Wada H. et.al. Redox status of coenzyme q10 is associated with chronological age. JAGS July 2007 Vol. 55 No. 7

9. Folkers K. Survey on the vitamin aspects of coenzyme Q. Int J Vitam Res.1969;39:334-352.

10. Langsjoen PH, Langsjoen AM. Biofactors, 2003: 18(1-4); 101-11.

11. Sinatra S, The Coenzyme Q10 Phenomenon. McGraw-Hill Professional, 1998

12. Langsjoen, PH, M.D., F.A.C.C. Introduction To Coenzyme Q10. Available at; http://faculty.washington.edu/ely/coenzq10.html

13. Crane FL: The natural occurrence of coenzyme Q and related compounds. J Biol Chem 234:2169–2175, 1959.

14. Dutton PL, Ohnishi T, Darrouzet E, Leonard, MA, Sharp RE, Cibney BR, Daldal F and Moser CC. 4 Coenzyme Q oxidation reduction reactions in mitochondrial electron transport (pp 65-82) in Coenzyme Q: Molecular mechanisms in health and disease edited by Kagan VE and Quinn PJ, CRC Press (2000), Boca Raton

15. Ernster L, Dallner G. Biochemical, physiological and medical aspects of ubiquinone function.Biochim-Biophys-Acta. 1995 May 24; 1271(1): 195-204

16. Arroyo, A, Navarro F, Gomez-Diaz C, Crane FL, Alcain FJ, Navas P, Villalba JM. Interactions between ascorbyl free radical and coenzyme Q at the plasma membrane. J Bioenergy Biomembr. 2000 Apr; 32(2):199-210

17. Frei B, Kim M, And Ames B. Ubiquinol-10 is an effective lipid-soluble antioxidant at physiological concentrations. Proc. Nati. Acad. Sci. USA. Vol. 87, pp. 4879-4883, June 1990. Medical Sciences

18. Langsjoen PH, Langsjoen AM. Supplemental Ubiquinol in patients with advanced congestive heart failure. Biofactors 32 (2008), 119-128.

19. Mae, T., Sakamoto, Y., Morikawa, S., Hidaka, T., 2001. Pharmaceutical composition comprising coenzyme Q10. US Patent, No. 6,184,255 B1

20. http://www.census.gov/popest/national/

21. http://www.census.gov/ipc/www/usinterimproj/

22. Greene DE and Vande Zande HD. Universal energy principle of biological systems and the unity of bioenergetics, Proceedings of the National Academy of Sciences of the United States of America, Vol. 78, Issue 9, September 1981, pp. 5344-5347.

23. Banerjee R. Redox Biochemistry. John Wiley and Sons, 2007

24. Ernster L, Dallner G. Biochemical, physiological and medical aspects of ubiquinone function. Biochim Biophys Acta, 1995;1271:195-204.

25. Mizuno K, Tanaka M, Nozaki S et al., Antifatigue effects of coenzyme Q10 during physical fatigue, Nutrition. Vol. 24, Issue 4, April 2008, pp. 293-9.

26. Cooke M, Iosia M, Buford T et al., Effects of acute and 14-day coenzyme Q10 supplementation on exercise performance in both trained and untrained individuals, Journal of the International Society of Sports Nutrition, March 4, 2008.

27. Somani SM, Arroyo CM. Exercise training generates ascorbate free radical in rat heart.Indian J Physiol Pharmacol. 1995 Oct;39(4):323-9.

28. http://www.connecticutcenterforhealth.com/coq10.html,

29. http://lpi.oregonstate.edu/infocenter/othernuts/coq10/#function

30. Baggio E, Gandini R, Plancher AC, Passeri M, Carmosino G. Italian multicenter study on the safety and efficacy of coenzyme Q10 as adjunctive therapy in heart failure (interim analysis). The CoQ10 Drug Surveillance Investigators. Clin Investig. 1993;71(8 Suppl):S145-9.

31. Lloyd-Jones D, et al. Heart Disease and Stroke Statistics--2009 Update. A Report From the American Heart Association Statistics Committee and Stroke Statistics Subcommittee. Circulation. 2008 Dec 15.

32. Folkers K., Vadhanavikit S., Mortensen S.A. (1985) Biochemical rationale and myocardial tissue data on the effective therapy of cardiomyopathy with coenzyme Q10. In: Proc. Natl. Acad. Sci., U.S.A., vol. 82(3), pp 901-904.

33. Folkers-K. Langsjoen-P. Langsjoen-P-H. Therapy with coenzyme Q10 of patients in heart failure who are eligible or ineligible for a transplant. Biochem-Biophys-Res-Commun. 1992 Jan 15. 182(1). P 247-53.

34. Langsjoen PH, Langsjoen AM. Overview of the use of CoQ10 in cardiovascular disease. BioFactors 1999 9:273-84. http://wwwcsi.unian.it/coenzymeQ/overview.html

35. Serebruan VI, Ordonez JV, Herzong WR, Rohde M, Mortensen SA, Folkers K, Gurbel PA. Dietary coenzyme q10 supplementation alters platelet size and inhibits human vironectin (CD51/CD61) receptor expression. J Cardiovasc Pharmacol. 1997; 29(1):16-22.

36. Langsjoen-P-H. Folkers-K. Lyson-K. Muratsu-K. Lyson- T. Langsjoen-P. Effective and safe therapy with coenzyme Q10 for cardiomyopathy. Klin-Wochenschr. 1988 Jul 1. 66(13). P 583-90.

37. Data from IMS Health, Annual Report on prescription drug trends (Feb 20, 2008). www.imshealth.com..

38. Devin Mann, MD, MS; Kristi Reynolds, PhD, MPH; Donald Smith, MD; Paul Muntner, PhD. Trends in Statin Use and Low-Density Lipoprotein Cholesterol Levels Among US Adults: Impact of the 2001 National Cholesterol Education Program Guidelines. The Annals of Pharmacotherapy, 11/2008. Trends in Statin Use in the Civilian Noninstitutionalized Medicare Population, 1997 and 2002," Statistical Brief #97, Agency for Healthcare Research and Quality (September 2005). Based on data from the Medicare Expenditure Panel Survey. www.ahrq.gov.

39. Peter H. Langsjoen, M.D., F.A.c.c. The clinical use of HMG CoA-reductase inhibitors (statins) and the associated depletion of the essential co-factor coenzyme Qlo; a review of pertinent human and animal data.

40. Dr. Julian M. Whitaker, M.D. Citizen Petition To Change The Labeling For All Statin Drugs . . . Recommending Use Of 100-200mg Per Day Of Supplemental Co-Enzyme Qlo (Including Cardiomyopathy And Congestive Heart Failure). To Reduce The Risk Of Statin-Induced Myopathies. May 24,2002 Petitioner: http://www.fda.gov/OHRMS/DOCKETS/dailys/02/May02/052902/02p-0244-cp00001-01-vol1.pdf

41. Baggio E., Gandini R., Plancher A.C., Passeri M., Carmosino G. Italian multicenter study on safety and efficacy of coenzyme Q10 adjunctive therapy in heart failure. In: Eighth International Symposium on Biomedical and Clinical Aspects of Coenzyme Q (1994) Littarru G.P., Battino M. , Folkers K. (Eds) The Molecular Aspects of Medicine, Vol. 15 (Supplement), pp S287-S294.

42. M. Lamperrico, S. Comis. Italian multicenter study on the efficacy and safety of coenzyme Qlo as adjuvant therapy in heart failure". Clin Investig (1993) 71:S 129-S 133

43. Langsjoen P, Langsjoen P, Willis R, Folkers K. Usefulness of coenzyme Q10 in clinical cardiology: a long-term study. Mol Aspects Med. 1994;15 Suppl: s165-175

44. Seppo Ylauml-Herttuala. Macrophages and Oxidized Low Density Lipoproteins in the Pathogenesis of Atherosclerosis. Annals of Medicine, Volume 23, Issue 5 1991

45. Mohr D, Bowry VW, Stocker R. Dietary supplementation with coenzyme Q10 results in increased levels of ubiquinol-10 within circulating lipoproteins and increased resistance of human low-density lipoprotein to the initiation of lipid peroxidation. Biochim Biophys Acta. 1992;1126(3):247-254.

46. Littarru GP, Tiano L. Mol Biotechnol. Bioenergetic and antioxidant properties of coenzyme q10: recent developments. 2007 Sep ;37 (1):31-7 17914161 (P,S,G,E,B)

47. http://www.americanheart.org/presenter.jhtml?identifier4621

48. Rosenfeldt FL, Haas SJ, Krum H, Hadj A, Ng K, Leong JY, Watts GF. Coenzyme Q10 in the treatment of hypertension: a meta-analysis of the clinical trials. J Hum Hypertens. 2007 Apr;21(4):297-306. Epub 2007 Feb 8.

49. Levien TL, Baker DE. Coenzyme Q10. Pharmacist's letter. Stockton, CA: Therapeutic Research Center, 1998;14(2):8-9.

50. Langseth L. Oxidants, antioxidants and disease prevention. Belgium, International Life Science Institute, 1996

51. Kamikawa T, Kobayashi A, Yamashita T, et al. Effects of coenzyme Q10 on exercise tolerance in chronic stable angina pectoris. Am J Cardiol 1985;56:247.

52. Makhija N, Sendasgupta C, Kiran U, Lakshmy R, Hote MP, Choudhary SK, Airan B, Abraham R.The role of oral coenzyme Q10 in patients undergoing coronary artery bypass graft surgery. J Cardiothorac Vasc Anesth. 2008 Dec;22(6):832-9.

53. W.V.Suzy, W.W.Stogsdill, K.Folkers. Myocardial preservation by therapy with coenzyme Q10 during heart surgery. Clinical Investigator 1993;71(8 Suppl):S155-61.

54. R. Nakamura, G.P. Littarru, K. Folkers, ER.G. Wilkinson Study of CoQ10-enzymes in gingiva from patients with periodontal disease and evidence for a deficiency of coenzyme Q10 Proc. Natl. Acad. Sci. USA. 71, n.4, 1456-1460, 1974.

55. Bioenergetics in clinical medicine. V. Adjunctive treatment of periodontal disease with coenzyme Q10. Res Commun Chem Pathol Pharmacol. 1976 Aug; 14 (4): 715-9).

56. Rozen TD, Oshinsky ML, et al. Open label trial of coenzyme Q10 as a migraine preventive. Cephalalgia. 2002 Mar; 22(2):137-41)

57. Hershey et al. Headache 2007; 47:73-80).

58. Alleva, R., A. Scararmucci, et al. (1997). The Protective Role of Ubiquinol-10 Against Formation of Lipid Hydroperoxides in Human Seminal Fluid. Mol Aspects Med 18 Suppl: S221-8).

59. Khan M, et al. A pilot clinical trial of the effects of coenzyme Q10 on chronic tinnitus aurium. Otolaryngol Head Neck Surg. 2007 Jan;136(1):72-7).

60. Folkers K, et al. Research on Coenzyme Q10 in Clinical Medicine and Immunomodulation. Drugs Exp.Clin. Res. 11 (8), 539-545 (1985).

61. Ely JTA, Krone CA. A brief update on ubiquinone (Coenzyme Q10). J Orthomolecular Medicine 2000; 15(2):63-68. J Orthomolecular Medicine.

62. The Free Radical Theory of Aging, Antioxid Redox Signal. 2003 Oct; 5(5):557-61

63. Hoppe U, Bergemann J, Diembeck W, Ennen J, Gohla S, Harris I, Jacob J, Kielholz J, Mei W, Pollet D, Schachtschabel D, Sauermann G, Schreiner V, Stäb F, Steckel F. Coenzyme Q10, a cutaneous antioxidant and energizer. Biofactors. 1999;9(2-4):371-8

64. Quiles JL, Ochoa JJ, Huertas JR, Mataix J (2004). "Coenzyme Q supplementation protects from age-related DNA double-strand breaks and increases lifespan in rats fed on a PUFA-rich diet.". Exp Gerontol. 39 (2): 189–94.

65. http://www.icqa.org/Summary/FAQ.html

66. Pharmacotherapy 21(7):797-806, 2001. © 2001 Pharmacotherapy Publications

67. Hosoe K et al. / Regulatory Toxicology and Pharmacology 47 (2007) 19–28